THE PALEO KID'S
chocolate

27 Chocolate Lover Recipes
(Primal Gluten Free Kids Cookbook)

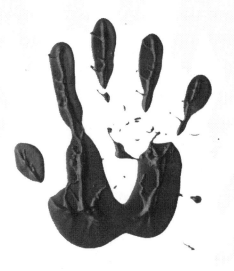

Kate Evans Scott

KL PRESS

DISCLAIMER

Although the author and publisher have made every effort to ensure that the information in this book was correct at press time, the author and publisher do not assume and hereby disclaim any liability to any party for any loss, damage, or disruption caused by errors or omissions, whether such errors or omissions result from negligence, accident, or any other cause.

This book is not intended as a substitute for the medical advice of physicians. The reader should regularly consult a physician in matters relating to his/her health and particularly with respect to any symptoms that may require diagnosis or medical attention.

This book is dedicated to my two beautiful children.

ACKNOWLEDGMENTS

Thank You to my friends and family for your encouragement. Your support has been the cornerstone of this creative process.

A special thanks also goes out to you the reader ~ I am grateful to be sharing this journey to health and happiness together with you.

CONTENTS

THE PALEO CHOCOLATE LOVER

If you or your kids are chocolate lovers, don't fret. You don't have to give up chocolate to live a Paleo lifestyle. It's not the actual cocoa in the chocolate that's unhealthy. The chocolates commonly found at the grocery stores, in the vending machines, and at the bakery are unhealthy because of the fats, sugars, and refined grains in them... not because of cocoa.

A small amount of dark chocolate is good for your heart. The flavonoids present in the skin of the cocoa bean are incredible for your circulatory system. They loosen up platelets and expand the arterial walls. Dark chocolate helps decrease our blood pressure and prevent arteriosclerosis.

Dark chocolate is a mood enhancer. Yep, dark chocolate helps you release the endorphins and serotonin that mimics the same rush of feelings you have when you're falling in love. Why do you think we give each other chocolate on Valentine's Day and first dates?

Dark chocolate helps your immune system. Dark chocolate is high in antioxidants, the immune system's free-radical sweepers. They help eradicate the harmful intruders that cause everything from allergies to colds to cancer.

A BRIEF HISTORY OF CHOCOLATE

The Aztec and Mayan cultures of Central America were the first known people to cultivate the seed of the cacao nut, grinding it and mixing it with spices to create a rich chocolate drink. This was around 2,000 BCE. They actually thought that the cacao plant was a gift from the gods, raising it up to the status of a precious gem. One king was actually served the sweet chocolate drink every day from a golden goblet.

Since then, chocolate has made its way into many cultures worldwide. It was brought to Europe by Christopher Columbus on his return voyage from the Americas, but it took about twenty years for the deliciousness of chocolate to capture the attention of society.

The mass production of chocolate and its subsequent hold on popular culture happened with the inception of Hershey's and Nestle, the two biggest chocolate producers in the world. The Swiss learned how to create a chocolate that perfectly balanced cacao and milk, leading eventually to the Nestle Company. Hershey was born in Pennsylvania, and the company sold one million dollars worth of chocolate in the early 1900s.

Now there is chocolate everywhere, from our café mochas to the chocolate bars in the vending machines at schools, work places, train stations, and elsewhere. We have chocolate cakes and cupcakes, chocolate chip cookies in our lunches, and milk shakes with our burgers. Well, as Paleo people, we avoid these sugar and fat-laden "treats." But that doesn't mean we have to forego the virtues of a gift from the gods. Not all chocolate is created equal.

EXTRA DARK CHOCOLATE AND HOMEMADE PALEO CHOCOLATE

There are some fantastic extra dark chocolates out there that have just small amounts of sugar and no dairy or gluten. Make sure the chocolate you choose is 80% cocoa or higher, ensuring you get all of the health benefits of the cacao with very little of the negatives from sugar and fat. If you want to keep the refined sugars out completely, use the recipe in this book as your jumping point -- your base chocolate for all the delicious recipes in the following pages.

"Enjoy Life" makes a low sugar, gluten free dark chocolate that most Paleo people feel is acceptable. You can find Enjoy Life at most health food stores and can order it online. Check your local health food store for other extra dark chocolate alternatives.

TOO MUCH OF A GOOD THING?

Yes, I'm giving you and your family the go-ahead to eat these decadent sweet treats... but not all the time. These should still be considered treats. Maybe a sundae on Sunday, or a cupcake to celebrate a special event. They shouldn't be eaten daily because they are still high in calories from honey, maple syrup, dried fruits and nuts.

You especially want to carefully monitor your consumption of "dessert" items if you are on the Paleo diet to lose weight. Make it a treat, and it will be all that much sweeter. Now go ahead... indulge!

"If there's no chocolate in Heaven, I'm not going."
— Jane Seabrook

Basic Paleo Chocolate

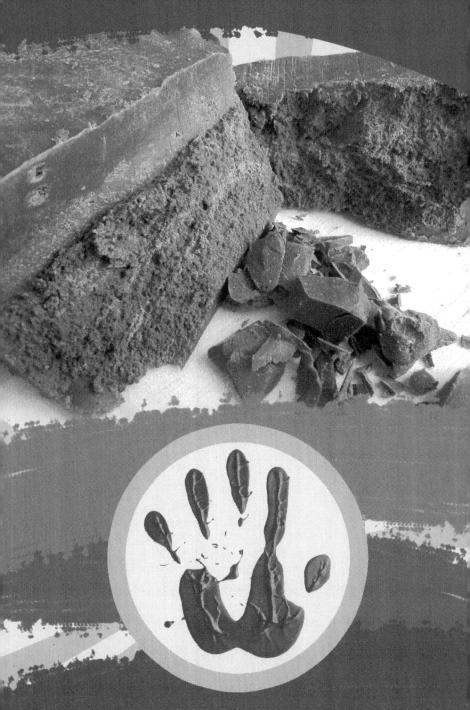

BASIC PALEO CHOCOLATE RECIPE

Paleo chocolate is really easy to make, and it's absolutely delicious...
especially if you're a fan of dark chocolate. If you're planning on doing
a bunch of baking, you can make a big hunk of chocolate for chunking
up. But if you just want some straight-up chocolate to feed your craving,
make it on a waxed paper lined cookie sheet or pour into chocolate
molds and eat it plain.

Ingredients:

- 1 cup cold-pressed coconut oil
- 1 cup raw cocoa powder
- ½ cup raw honey (or to taste)
- Dash of sea salt

Directions: In a heavy pot, melt the coconut oil. Whisk in the cocoa powder,
honey, and salt until everything is smooth and melted. Pour the melted chocolate
into a waxed paper lined pan or directly into chocolate molds.

Refrigerate or freeze for at least one hour or until set. Store in the refrigerator
until ready to use.

*If you want to reduce the calorie count and make a firmer chocolate with a crisp
break, replace the honey with liquid stevia extract.

Serving Size: ¼ cup   Yields: About 10 Servings
Prep Time: 2 min   Cook Time: 3 min   Total Time: 65 min

FROZEN CHOCOLATE TREATS

Banana Nibs

~

Chocolate Macadamia Pudding Pops

~

Almond Butter Cup Ice Cream

~

Vanilla Ice Cream Sundae

Banana Nibs

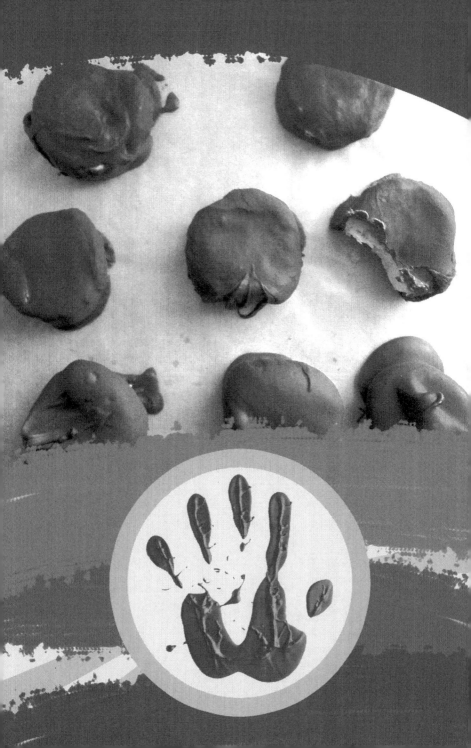

BANANA NIBS RECIPE

These are a summer go-to when our house is teaming with neighborhood kids. Free of all of the common allergens (peanuts, dairy, wheat, food dyes, eggs), we keep a batch of banana nibs in the freezer for quick treats. Plus I feel good about it, because there's fruit in every bite!

Ingredients:

- ½ cup Paleo chocolate or Enjoy Life chocolate chips
- 1 banana

Directions: Line a small pan or plate with waxed paper.

If your chocolate has already been set, melt it over low heat in a small pot, stirring constantly until JUST melted. *If using Enjoy Life chocolate chips, you may want to add ½ tsp of coconut oil to help it melt smoother. Pour the chocolate into a cup for easier dipping and allow to cool slightly to thicken.

Peel the banana and slice into ½" bite sizes. Place a slice into a small spoon and dunk it into the chocolate. Turn to coat. Lay the banana slice onto the waxed paper. Repeat until the entire banana has been used. Freeze on the tray for at least one hour or until frozen through.

Store remaining banana nibs in an airtight container in the freezer for up to two weeks.

Serving Size: 1/3 banana   Yields: 3 servings
Prep Time: 10 min   Total Time: 70 minutes

Chocolate Macadamia Pudding Pops

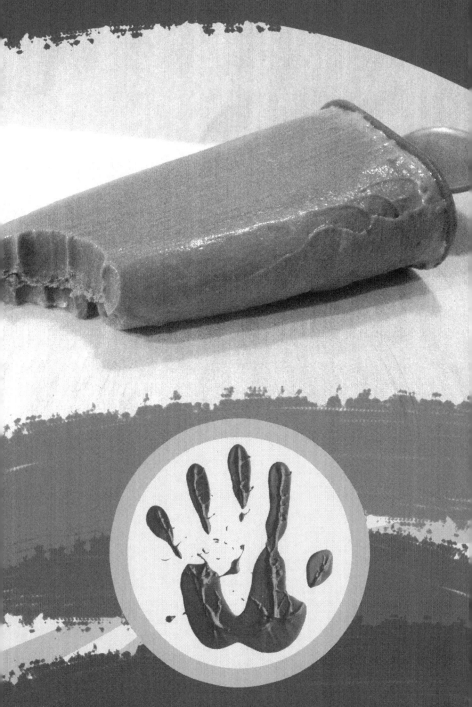

CHOCOLATE MACADAMIA PUDDING POPS RECIPE

Pudding pops are a classic childhood favorite, and these honestly taste even better than the ones I remember from my youth. Four ingredients, blended to a creamy perfection, make these freezer treats as easy as... pudding!

Ingredients:

- 1 cup raw macadamia nuts, soaked over night
- 1/3 cup cocoa powder
- ¼ cup honey (or to taste)
- 1 tsp vanilla extract

Directions: Rinse the soaked macadamia nuts. Place all ingredients into your high-powered kitchen blender and process until smooth and creamy. Pour the mixture into store-bought popsicle makers or small paper cups until just below the rim. Insert the handles or popsicle sticks. Freeze for at least four hours.

To remove the pop from the popsicle mold, gently run the base under warm water until the pudding pop releases easily.

Serving Size: 1 pudding pop
Yields: 2 to 4 pops depending on popsicle maker size
Prep Time: Overnight + 4 hrs, 10 min
Total Time: Overnight + 4 hrs, 10 minutes

Almond Butter Cup
Ice Cream

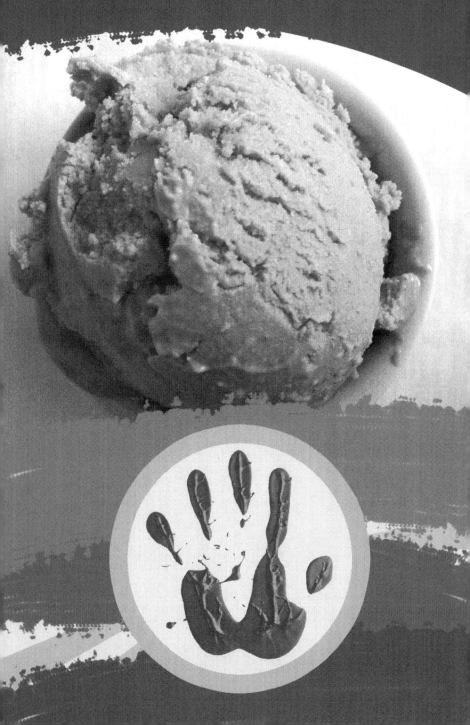

ALMOND BUTTER CUP
ICE CREAM RECIPE

One of the best investments you can make in your Paleo kitchen is an ice cream maker, especially if you have kids (or kid-like adults) in your house! You can pick up a small counter top unit for less than $40 at some big box stores. This mock peanut butter cup ice cream is one of our favorites, but the possibilities are as broad as your imagination! (**Note:** ice cream maker needed)

Ingredients:

- 1 14oz can full fat coconut milk
- 1/3 cup cocoa powder
- ¼ cup creamy almond butter, softened
- ¼ - ½ pure maple syrup (to taste)
- 1 tsp vanilla extract
- Pinch sea salt

Directions: Place all ingredients, except almond butter, in the bowl of your kitchen mixer with whisk attachment. Mix until smooth. Gently stir in the almond butter. Freeze according to your ice cream maker's manufacturer directions.

Serve immediately or store in an airtight container in the freezer up to two weeks. Thaw slightly before serving.

Serving Size: ½ cup   Yields: 4 servings   Prep Time: 5 min
Freeze Time: about 30 min   Total Time: 35 min

Vanilla Ice Cream Sundae

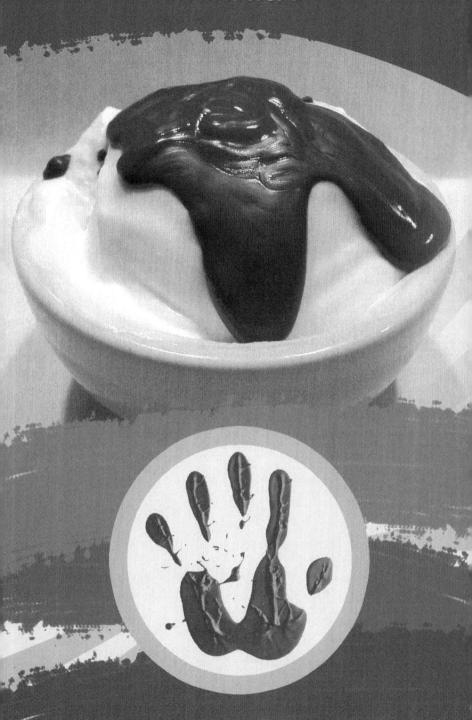

VANILLA ICE CREAM SUNDAE RECIPE

Do you remember walking up to the ice cream shop and ordering a vanilla cone dunked in chocolate? The coating hardens, you bite in and the ice cream dribbles down your arm. If you loved that cone, then this dessert is for you... minus the sticky arm. (**Note:** ice cream maker needed)

Ingredients for the ice cream:

- 1 14 oz can full fat coconut milk
- 1 egg yolk
- ¼ cup raw honey, softened
- 1 tsp pure vanilla extract

Ingredients for the chocolate:

- ½ cup Enjoy Life chocolate chips
- 1 tbsp coconut oil

Directions: Whisk together the ice cream ingredients until well blended. Freeze according to your ice cream maker's manufacturer directions.

In a small pot or double boiler set over low heat, melt the chocolate chips with the coconut oil. When the ice cream is completely frozen, scoop into four bowls. Drizzle with the chocolate sauce and allow the chocolate to harden into a shell.

Serving Size: ½ cup   Yields: 4 servings   Prep Time: 10 min
Freeze Time: about 30 min   Total Time: 40 min

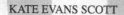

PUDDING, PIES AND FRUITS

Cashew Chocolate Pudding

~

Chocolate Coconut Cream Pie

~

Chocolate Chip Cheesecake Squares

~

Chocolate Dipped Strawberries

~

Dark Chocolate Raw Truffles

~

Easy Chocolate Raspberry Cups

~

Fig And Cacao Nib Power Bars

~

No-Bake Cookies

Cashew Chocolate Pudding

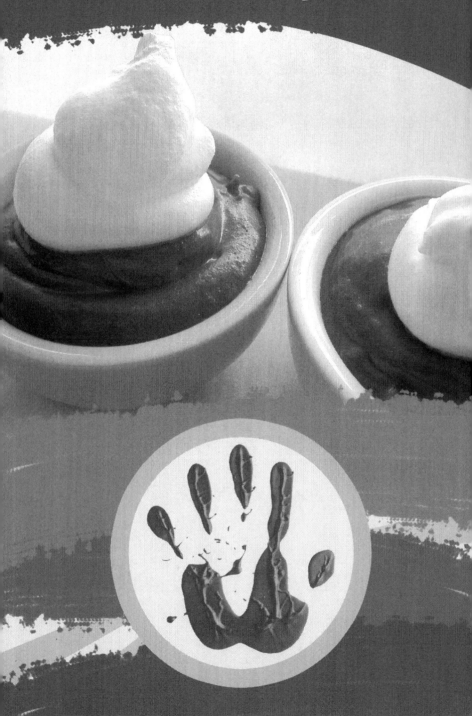

CASHEW CHOCOLATE PUDDING RECIPE

This pudding is so easy to make, you'll probably start whipping up a batch every day. Unlike the Paleo puddings that use banana or avocado, the cashew pudding holds up when packed in a lunch box or when frozen. Topped with a dollop of coconut whipped cream, they are the perfect sweet ending to any meal.

Ingredients:

- 1 cup raw cashews, soaked over night
- ¼ cup cocoa powder
- ¼ cup maple syrup
- 1 tsp vanilla extract
- Pinch of sea salt
- Dollop of coconut whipped cream (optional)

Directions: Place all ingredients into your high-powered kitchen blender. Blend until smooth. Serve immediately or refrigerate until ready to serve. Garnish with a dollop of coconut whipped cream.

Serving Size: ½ cup   Yields: 2 to 3 servings
Prep Time: Overnight + 5 min   Total Time: Overnight + 5 min

Chocolate Coconut Cream Pie

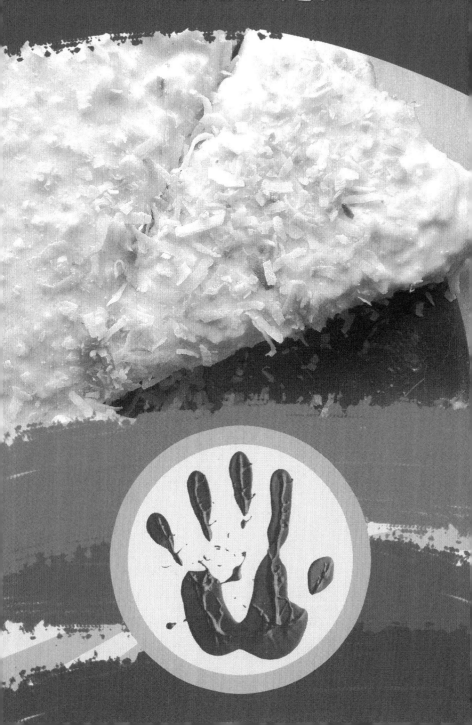

CHOCOLATE COCONUT CREAM PIE RECIPE

If you like coconut cream pie, you'll fall in love with this chocolate-layered version of the old classic. No baking. No custard making. This is almost fail-proof! Serve it at your next potluck and see if anyone notices that it's a raw, healthy dessert!

Ingredients for the crust:

- 1 cup raw almonds
- ½ cup medjool dates, packed
- 1 tbsp coconut oil
- ½ tsp cinnamon
- Dash salt

Ingredients for the chocolate layer:

- 2 recipes Cashew Chocolate Pudding (see recipe)
- Ingredients for the coconut layer:
- 2 14oz cans full fat coconut milk (Yields about 1 cup cream)
- ¾ cup shredded unsweetened coconut, divided
- 1 ½ tsp pure vanilla extract
- 2 tbsp raw honey, softened

Directions: THE NIGHT BEFORE: Put the cans of coconut into the refrigerator upside down. Soak the cashews according to the Cashew Chocolate Pudding recipe.

For the crust: Place all of the crust ingredients into the food processor and process until a ball forms, about four minutes. The texture will be grainy. Press the crust into the bottom and slightly up the sides of a 9" or 10" springform pan. Set aside.

Prepare the Cashew Chocolate Pudding according to recipe instructions. Spread the double-batch of pudding evenly onto the prepared crust. Heat the oven to 350°F. Spread ¼ cup of the shredded coconut onto a pan and toast for about ten minutes, or until just golden brown. Remove from oven and let cool.

Flip the cold coconut milk cans right side up and puncture two holes in each can with a can opener. Pour out the liquid. (You can save this! Coconut milk, yum!) Open the lid entirely and what you have left is coconut cream.

Scoop the coconut cream into a large mixing bowl. Whisk in the vanilla extract and softened honey. Keep whisking until the mixture is getting fluffy. Stir in ½ cup shredded coconut. Spread this mixture evenly over the top of the chocolate pudding layer. Sprinkle with toasted coconut and refrigerate at least one hour.

Serving Size: 1 slice   Yields: 8 servings

Prep Time: Overnight + 1 Hour, 25 min   Total Time: Overnight + 1 Hour, 25 min

Chocolate Chip Cheesecake Squares

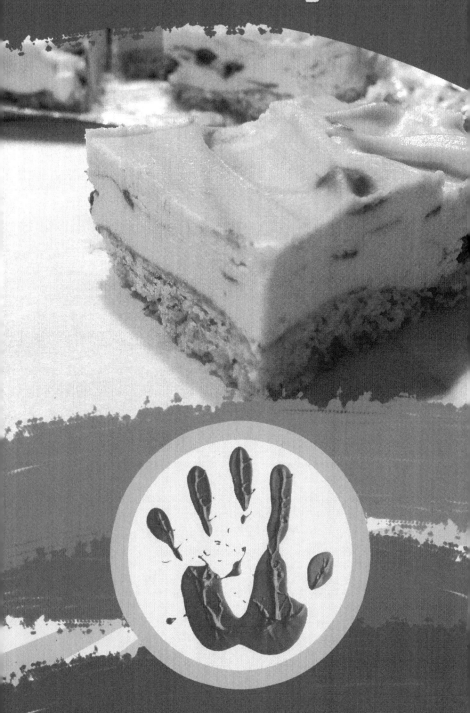

CHOCOLATE CHIP CHEESECAKE SQUARES RECIPE

This cheesecake is so tangy and creamy that you wouldn't believe there's no cream cheese in it if you hadn't made it yourself! The trick is soaked cashews. This is a step you absolutely cannot skip, so plan a day ahead. After a night of sitting in a water bath, these little nuts turn into silky delights and take on any flavor you add to them.

Crust Ingredients:

- 1 cup almond meal
- 3 tbsp coconut oil
- 1 tbsp pure maple syrup
- Pinch of sea salt and cinnamon

Filling Ingredients:

- 2 cups raw cashews
- ½ cup lemon juice
- ¼ cup coconut oil
- ¼ cup raw honey, softened
- 1 tsp vanilla extract
- ½ cup Enjoy Life dark chocolate chips

Directions: THE NIGHT BEFORE — Place the cashews in a bowl and cover completely with cold water. Cover and let soak overnight. Preheat oven to 325°F.

In a small bowl, mix together the crust ingredients and press into the bottom of a 9" x 9" glass baking dish. Bake for 15 minutes or until the crust is golden and set. Remove from oven and cool completely.

To make the filling: Rinse the cashews with cold water and drain. Place all filling ingredients, except chocolate chips, in your high-powered kitchen blender and process on high until smooth. Gently stir in the chocolate chips.

Pour filling in an evenly layer over cooled crust. Cover and freeze at least one hour. Remove from refrigerator ½ hour before serving. Cut into squares and enjoy.

Serving Size: 1 square   Yields: 16 servings
Prep Time: Overnight + 20 min   Bake Time: 15 min
Total: Overnight + 45 min

Chocolate Dipped Strawberries

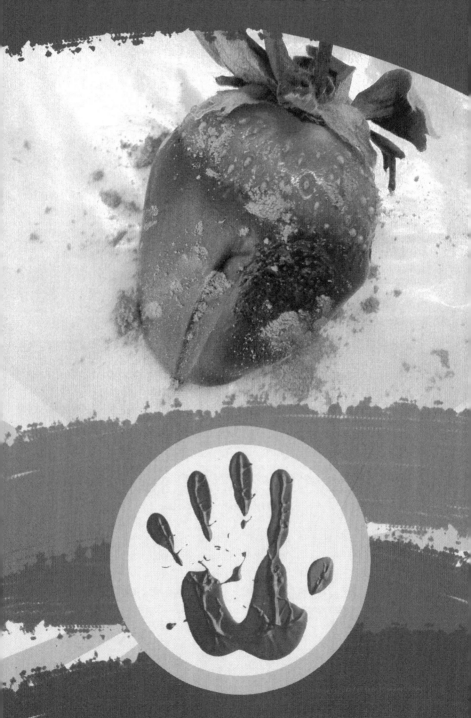

CHOCOLATE DIPPED STRAWBERRIES RECIPE

Life, and dessert, couldn't get simpler. Fresh strawberries dipped in pure dark chocolate are a healthy favorite for any gathering or summer afternoon snack. Have the kids help you make these, even the littlest ones. There is really no way to make a mistake and they'll be proud to share their culinary success! Tip: Use chilled strawberries to help the chocolate harden quicker.

Ingredients:

- 12 large ripe strawberries
- ¾ cup dark chocolate, Paleo chocolate, or Enjoy Life chocolate chips

Directions: Wash and dry the strawberries, leaving leaves intact. Lay a sheet of waxed paper on a tray or plate.

Melt the chocolate in a small pot set over low heat, stirring regularly, until chocolate is just melted. Pour chocolate into a short mug (making dipping easier). If the chocolate is very runny, as the Paleo chocolate might be, allow it to cool slightly before dipping.

Holding a strawberry carefully by the stem/leaves, dunk it into the chocolate. Let it drip off before laying the dipped strawberry on its side on the waxed paper. Repeat until all of the strawberries have been used.

Allow the chocolate to harden before serving. Keep in an airtight container in the refrigerator up to two days.

Serving Size: 3 strawberries   Yields: 4 servings
Prep Time: 15 min   Total Time: 15 min

Dark Chocolate Raw Truffles

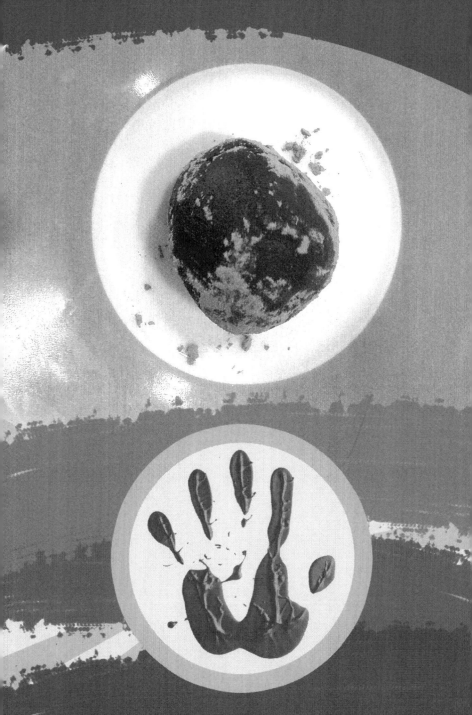

DARK CHOCOLATE RAW TRUFFLE RECIPE

Truffles in minutes? You can do it. These are especially great when you're running late for a potluck, have unexpected guests, or when you just need a bite of chocolate to maintain your sanity!

Ingredients:

- 1 ½ cups raw almonds
- 1 cup medjool dates
- ¼ cup cocoa powder
- 1 tsp pure vanilla extract
- Pinch sea salt
- Cocoa powder for dusting

Directions: Place the almonds, dates, cocoa powder, vanilla, and sea salt in the food processor. Process until smooth and the dough clumps into a ball.

Pull small chunks of dough off of the ball and roll until a smooth truffle ball forms. Roll the truffle in cocoa powder, shredded coconut, or crushed nuts. Store in the refrigerator in an airtight container up to ten days.

Serving Size: 3 truffles   Yields: 10 servings
Prep Time: 10 min   Total Time: 10 min

Easy Chocolate Raspberry Cups

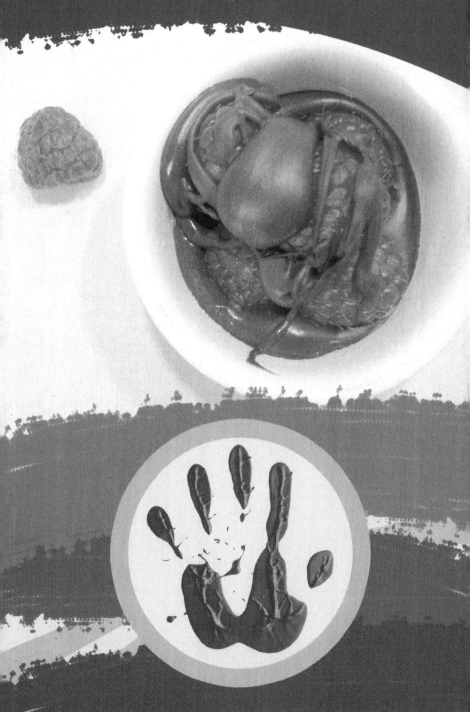

EASY CHOCOLATE RASPBERRY CUP RECIPE

Raspberries and chocolate are a match made in heaven. You only need two ingredients for this recipe—chocolate and raspberries. If you have some little dip-cups, these desserts look beautiful on a tray as a fancy petit dessert for parties.

Ingredients:

- 20 fresh raspberries
- 4 tbsp homemade chocolate or Enjoy Life dark chocolate chips

Directions: Wash and dry the raspberries, taking care not to squish them. If you are just making the chocolate, skip the cooling step. If you are using prepared chocolate, place the chocolate in a small pot set over very low heat. Stir constantly until just melted.

Place ½ tbsp. chocolate into each of four small dipping cups. Pile five raspberries in each cup. Drizzle ½ tbsp. chocolate on top of each raspberry pile. Serve immediately or allow to cool for a hardened chocolate dessert. Serve with tiny petit spoons.

Serving Size; 1   Yields: 4 servings
Prep Time: 10 min   Total Time: 10 min

Fig and Cacao Nib Power Bars

FIG AND CACAO NIB POWER BAR RECIPE

Raw cacao nibs are packed with vitamins and minerals. They're a super antioxidant as well. Crunchy and chocolatey with the slight wine after-note, they will certainly give your morning power bar an awesome punch.

Ingredients:

- 10 dried figs
- 1 cup raw almonds
- 1 tsp vanilla extract
- Pinch sea salt
- ¼ cup raw cacao nibs

Directions: Cover the figs in water and soak for 15 minutes. Drain. Place the figs, almonds, vanilla, and sea salt into the food processor and process until a dough ball forms. Add the cacao nibs and process until mixed.

Remove the dough ball to a sheet of waxed paper. Using your hands, press the dough into a rectangle about ½" thick. Cut into five "bars." Wrap in waxed paper and store up to one week in a zip-top bag.

Serving Size: 1 bar   Yields: 5 servings
Prep Time: 20 min   Total Time: 20 min

No-Bake Cookies

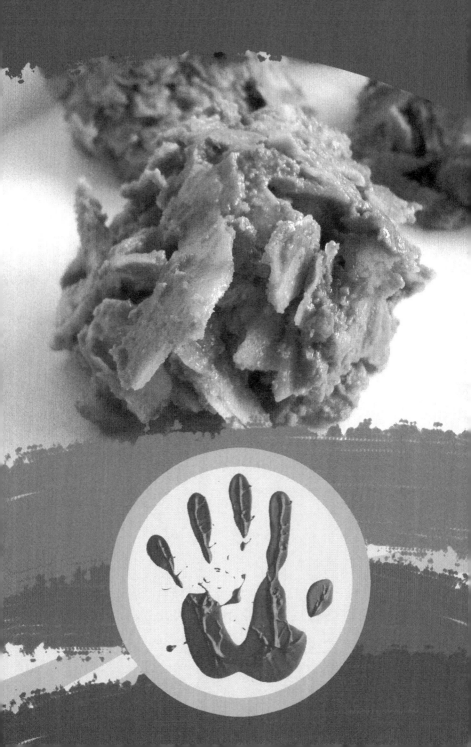

NO-BAKE COOKIES RECIPE

Remember no-bake cookies as a kid? Oats, peanut butter, and chocolate melted in a pot and then dropped in little mounds onto waxed paper? This is your cookie again. Embrace your inner child.

Ingredients:

- 3 cups flaked unsweetened coconut
- 1 cup smooth sunflower seed butter (or nut butter)
- 3 tbsp raw honey
- 2 tbsp coconut oil
- 1 tsp vanilla extract

Directions: Place the sunflower seed butter, raw honey, coconut oil, and vanilla extract in a small pot set over low heat. Heat the ingredients slowly, stirring regularly, until the mixture is slightly melted. Stir in the coconut.

Drop by the spoonful onto waxed paper and allow to cool completely, about twenty minutes. Store in an airtight container up to three days.

Serving Size: 1 cookie   Yields: about 12 servings
Prep Time: 15 min   Cool Time: 20 min   Total Time: 35 min

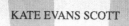

BAKED GOODS

Chocolate Chunk Sheet Cake

~

Chewy Almond Brownies

~

Chocolate Granola

~

Chocolate Chip Banana Bread

~

Two Minute Mug Cake

~

Chocolate Cupcakes

~

Crisp Chocolate Chip Cookies

~

NOreo Cream Cookies

~

Chocolate Striped Macaroons

Chocolate Chunk
Sheet Cake

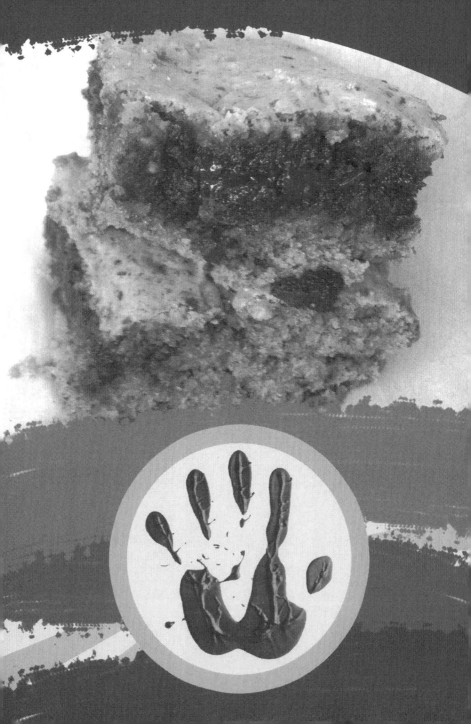

CHOCOLATE CHUNK
SHEET CAKE RECIPE

This sheet cake is soft, moist, and delicious even without any kind of icing. Have it for breakfast, pack it into a lunch box, or just grab a slice right out of the pan.

Ingredients:

- 1 cup almond butter
- 1 cup almond meal
- 3 eggs
- ½ cup chocolate chunks (Paleo homemade or 80% cocoa dark chocolate)
- 1 tsp vanilla extract
- 1 tsp baking soda
- Dash salt
- Coconut oil for greasing

Directions: Preheat oven to 350°F.

Grease a 9"x 9" square baking pan with coconut oil. Set aside.

Place all remaining ingredients, except chocolate, into the bowl of your kitchen mixer. Mix with the regular attachment until everything is well blended. Stir in the chocolate chunks and pour batter into the prepared pan.

Bake at 350°F for about thirty minutes or until the cake bounces back when depressed.

Serving Size: 1 slice   Yields: 12 servings
Prep Time: 10 min   Bake Time: 30 min   Total Time: 40 min

Chewy Almond Brownies

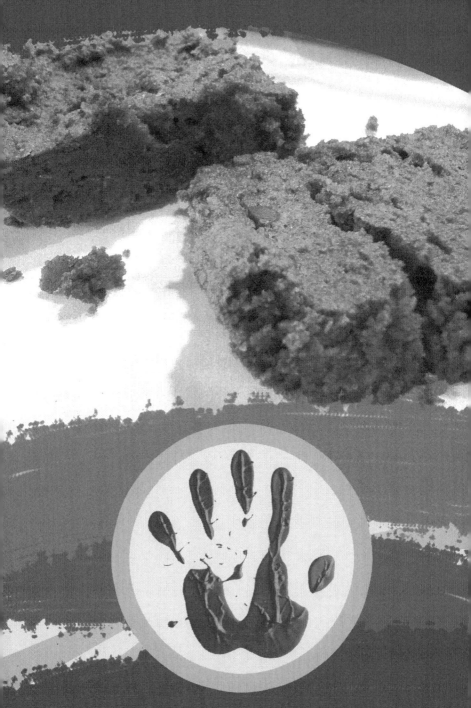

CHEWY ALMOND BROWNIES RECIPE

Every chocolate lover is passionate about brownies. This recipe for soaked almond brownies fooled the palate of my most skeptical friend. Pure maple syrup is the perfect sweetener complement to the dark, gooey, nutty chocolate in this simple recipe.

Ingredients:

- 2 cups raw almonds, soaked overnight
- ½ cup grass fed butter or coconut oil, plus some for greasing pan
- 2 eggs
- ¾ cup raw cocoa powder
- ½ cup pure maple syrup
- 1 tsp vanilla extract
- ½ tsp sea salt
- ¼ cup Enjoy Life chocolate chips

Directions: THE NIGHT BEFORE — Place the almonds in a bowl and cover with cold water. Cover and soak overnight.

Preheat oven to 350°F. Lightly grease a 6" x 11" glass baking pan. Set aside.

Rinse and drain the soaked almonds. Place them in your high powered kitchen blender with the butter, eggs, maple syrup, cocoa powder, vanilla and sea salt. Process until smooth. Gently mix in the chocolate chips and pour the batter into the prepared pan.

Bake about 40 minutes or until the brownies are set and pulling a bit away from the pan edges. Cool in the pan.

Serving Size: 1 brownie   Yields: 16 servings
Prep Time: Overnight + 10 min   Bake Time: 40 min
Total Time: Overnight + 50 min

Chocolate
Granola

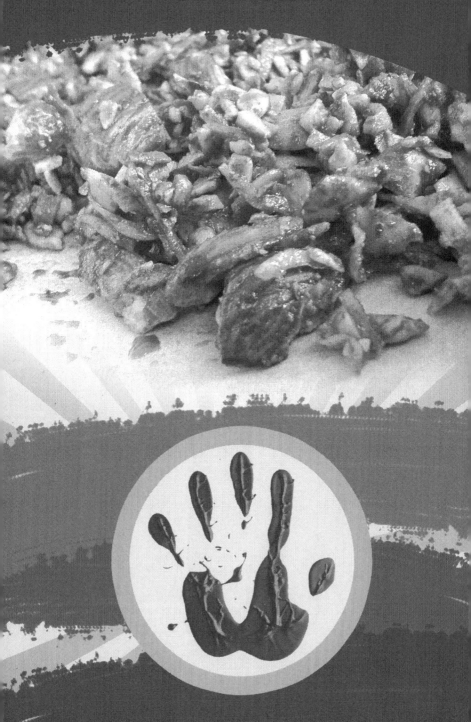

CHOCOLATE GRANOLA RECIPE

Chocolate for breakfast? Yes, please. Paleo granola is really simple to prepare, and with a healthy dose of cocoa powder it's a real morning treat! Pour it over coconut yogurt or eat like cereal with almond milk.

Ingredients:

- 1 cup raw almonds
- 1 cup unsweetened shredded coconut
- ½ cup pepitos
- ½ cup unsalted sunflower seeds
- ¼ cup raw honey, melted
- 2 tbsp melted coconut oil
- 2 tbsp cocoa powder
- ½ tsp salt

Directions: Preheat oven to 250°F.

Place the almonds, coconut, pepitos, and sunflower seeds in the food processor and pulse several times until the nuts and seeds are chopped into chunks. Add remaining ingredients and pulse several times until everything is well mixed.

Line a jellyroll pan with parchment paper and pour the granola mixture on it in an even layer. Bake for about two hours, stirring every half hour. Let the granola cool in the pan. It will harden and get crunchy as it cools.

Once completely cooled, you can store it in an airtight container for up to two weeks.

Serving Size: ½ cup   Yields: 8 servings   Prep Time: 10 min
Bake Time: 2 hours   Total Time: 2 hours, 10 min

Chocolate Chip
Banana Bread

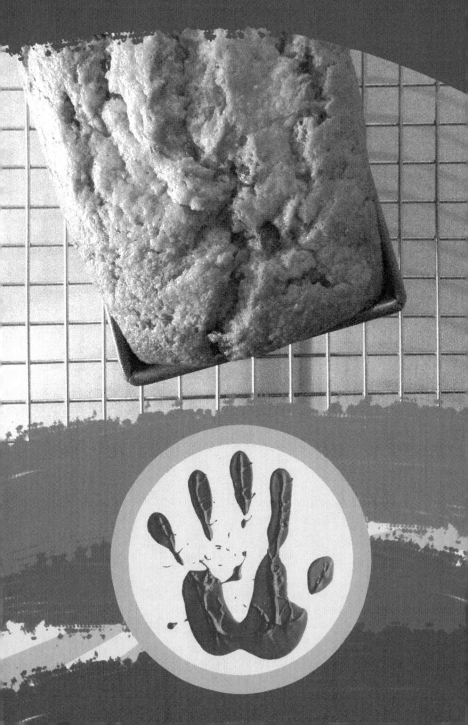

CHOCOLATE CHIP BANANA BREAD RECIPE

If you want to convert a traditionalist to the Paleo way of life, serve them this bread. It has to be one of the most delicious things I've ever put into my mouth. Serve it plain or slathered in butter or NOTella. Any way you slice it; this bread will be gobbled right up.

Ingredients:

- 1 ½ almond meal
- ½ cup almond butter
- ½ cup pure maple syrup
- 4 tbsp coconut oil (melted), plus extra for greasing
- 3 ripe bananas, mashed
- 3 large eggs
- 1 ½ tsp baking powder (gluten free)
- 1 tsp vanilla extract
- ½ cups chocolate chips
- ½ tsp salt

Directions: Preheat oven to 350°F. Grease a 4"x 9" (standard size) loaf pan with coconut oil.

In a large mixing bowl, beat together the eggs, almond butter, maple syrup, mashed bananas, and vanilla extract. In a separate bowl, mix together the almond meal, and sea salt. Add the almond meal mixture to the egg mixture and beat until smooth. Fold in the chocolate chips.

Pour the batter evenly into the pan. Bake for 55 – 65 minutes or until a toothpick inserted into the center comes out clean. Cool in pan for about ten minutes, and then transfer to a wire cooling rack to finish cooling.

Serving Size: 1 slice Yields: 8 Servings
Prep Time: 15 min Bake Time: 65 min
Total Time: 1 Hr, 20 min

Two Minute Mug Cake

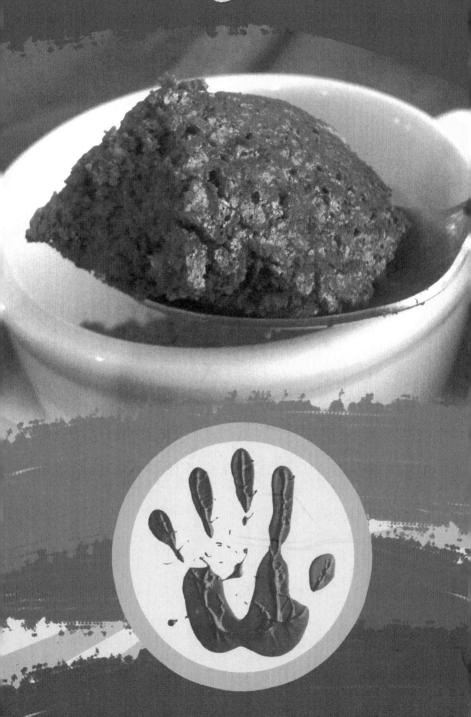

TWO MINUTE MUG CAKE RECIPE

Some of our Paleo friends use the microwave, some do not. If you do, this personal-sized dessert comes out hot and gooey in just two minutes. If you use the oven instead, don't worry. You only have to wait a few minutes longer to indulge in this lava-cake style chocolate goodness.

Ingredients:

- 1 egg
- 2 tbsp cocoa powder
- 3 tbsp almond meal
- 2 tbsp pure maple syrup
- 1 tsp pure vanilla extract

Directions: Place all ingredients in an oven or microwave safe mug or ramekin. Mix together well with a metal fork. Microwave, uncovered, for two minutes. Enjoy plain or with a dollop of coconut whipped cream or vanilla ice cream.

Alternately, preheat oven to 350°F. Bake the mixed cake in an ovenproof ramekin for about fifteen minutes.

Serving Size: 1 Mug Cake   Yields: 1 Serving   Prep Time: 2 minutes
Bake Time: 2 – 15 min   Total Time: 4 – 19 min

Chocolate Cupcakes

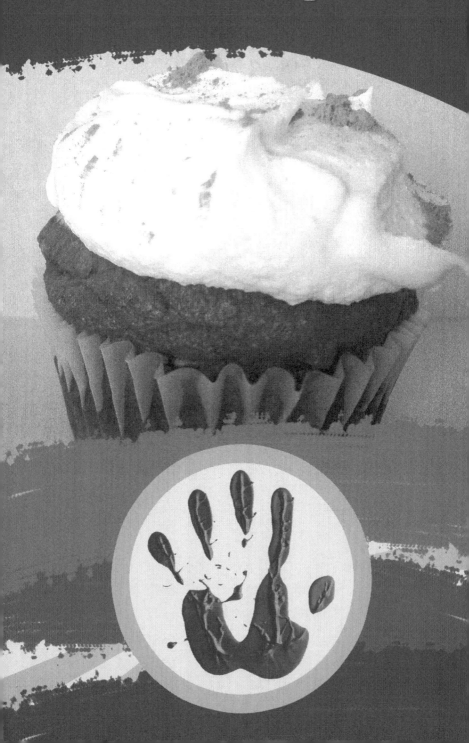

CHOCOLATE CUPCAKES WITH WHIPPED TOPPING RECIPE

The texture of this cupcake is light and fluffy with a crisp top and deep chocolate flavors. Top it with a dollop of coconut whipped cream, or spread with Chocolate Buttercream Frosting or NOTella. If you want one for breakfast, eat it plain... because muffins are just naked cupcakes, right?

Ingredients:

- 1 ½ cups cashew meal
- 1 cup mashed banana
- 2 large eggs
- ½ cup cashew butter
- ½ cup pure maple syrup
- 4 tbsp grassfed butter
- 1/3 cup cocoa powder
- 1 ½ tsp baking powder
- 1 tsp vanilla extract
- ½ tsp sea salt

Directions: Preheat oven to 350°F.

Place all ingredients into the bowl of your standing mixer with the standard mixing attachment. Mix until the batter is uniform and fluffy. Fill twelve cupcake cups with paper liners.

Fill the cupcake liners ¾ full of batter and bake 35 – 40 minutes or until fluffy and crisp on top and a toothpick inserted into the center comes out clean. Cool in the pan and top with buttercream icing, NOTella, or a dollop of coconut whipped cream (pictured).

Serving Size: 1 cupcake   Yields: 12
Prep Time: 15 min   Bake Time: 40 min   Total Time: 55 min

Crisp Chocolate Chip Cookies

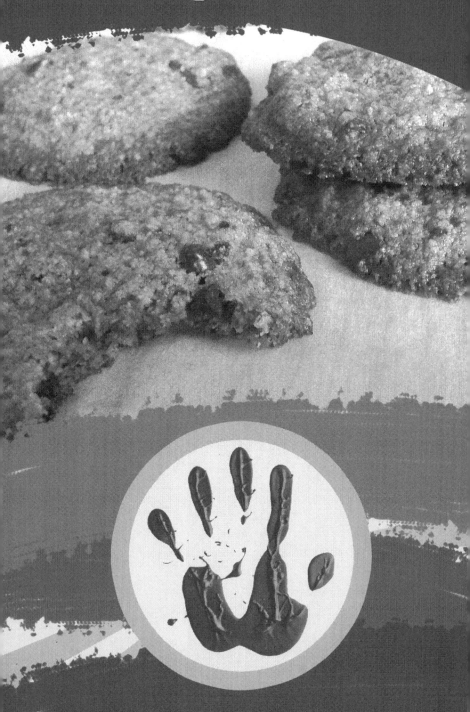

CRISP CHOCOLATE CHIP COOKIES RECIPE

Did you think you would never have a relationship with a crispy chocolate chip cookie again? Well, you will now. Unrefined coconut sugar bakes like refined cane sugar while retaining the vitamins and nutrients we all love about the coconut. So go ahead, fall in love with chocolate chip cookies all over again.

Ingredients:

- 2 cups almond flour
- 1 large egg
- ½ cup coconut oil, softened
- ¾ cup coconut sugar
- 1 tsp baking powder (gluten free)
- 1 tsp vanilla extract
- ½ tsp sea salt
- ½ cup Enjoy Life chocolate chips

Directions: Preheat oven to 350°F. Line a cookie sheet with parchment paper.

In a large mixing bowl, beat together the eggs, coconut sugar, coconut oil, and vanilla. In a separate bowl, mix together the almond flour, baking powder and sea salt. Add the almond mixture to the egg mixture and beat until well mixed.

Fold in the chocolate chips. Using a cookie scoop or a tablespoon, scoop the dough onto the parchment lined cookie sheet. Bake for about 10 minutes until the edges are golden. Cool on the sheet for a few minutes and then remove to a baking rack to finish cooling.

Serving Size: 1 cookie   Yields: About 20 servings
Prep Time: 10 min   Bake Time: 10 min   Total Time: 20 min

NOreo Cream Cookies

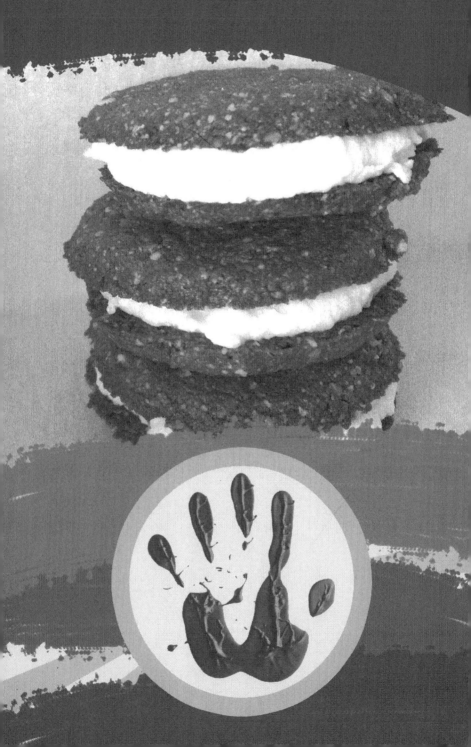

NOREO CREAM COOKIES RECIPE

This is not like the packaged, super-sweet, frosting-stuffed cookie in the blue packages. It's better! The cashew cookie is crunchy and chocolatey sandwiched around the creamy vanilla filling made with coconut butter. Grab a glass of almond milk, and twist, dunk, or munch. There's no one right way to eat a NOreo.

Ingredients:

- 2 cups cashew meal
- 3 tbsp coconut oil
- 2 tbsp raw honey
- 3 tbsp cocoa powder
- ½ tsp vanilla

Filling Ingredients:

- ½ cup coconut butter
- 2 tbsp raw honey, softened
- 3 tbsp coconut cream
- 1 tsp vanilla extract

Directions: Preheat the oven to 325°F.

Place all cookie ingredients in a large bowl and beat with electric beaters until a dough ball forms, about two minutes.

Pour the dough-ball out on a sheet of waxed paper and roll into a ¼" sheet. Using a round cookie cutter, cut circles until all dough has been used. Place the dough circles onto a parchment lined cookie sheet.

Bake rounds in the preheated oven for 12 – 15 minutes or until crisp. Allow to cool completely before filling.

To make the cream filling, place all ingredients into the food processor and pulse until smooth. Scoop the filling into the center of a cooled cookie, leaving space around the edge. Place the cookie "top" on and press gently until the filling comes to the edge of the cookie sandwich. Continue until all cookies have been used. Store in an airtight container up to five days.

Serving Size: 1 cookie   Yields: 8 servings
Prep Time: 20 min   Bake Time: 15 min   Total Time: 35 min

Chocolate Striped
Macaroons

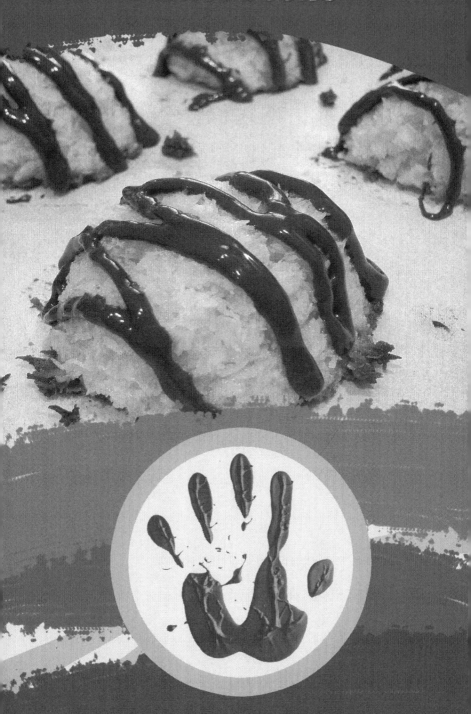

CHOCOLATE STRIPED MACAROONS RECIPE

Just a warning: These macaroons won't last long, so you'd better eat a few as soon as they're done cooling. The little two-bite treats are packed with soft, chewy deliciousness drizzled with the perfect touch of chocolate.

Ingredients:

- 1 ½ cups shredded unsweetened coconut
- 3 egg whites
- ¼ cup raw honey
- 1 tsp vanilla extract
- Pinch sea salt
- ¼ cup dark chocolate, homemade chocolate, or Enjoy Life chocolate chips (melted)

Directions: Preheat oven to 350°F. Line a cookie sheet with parchment paper.

In the bowl of your kitchen mixer, using the whisk attachment, beat the egg whites until stiff peaks form. Fold in the coconut, raw honey, vanilla, and sea salt.

Scoop the coconut mixture onto the parchment paper using a rounded tablespoon or cookie scoop. Bake for about twelve minutes or until the macaroons are golden brown. Cool on sheet.

Drizzle the melted chocolate onto the macaroons using a pastry bag with small tip, or just messy-dribble the chocolate! It all tastes great!

Serving Size: 1 macaroon   Yields: 12 servings
Prep Time: 10 min   Bake Time: 12 min   Total Time: 22 min

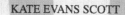

KATE EVANS SCOTT

TOPPINGS AND SPREADS

Chocolate Buttercream Frosting

~

Coconut Whipped Cream

~

NOTella

Chocolate Buttercream Frosting

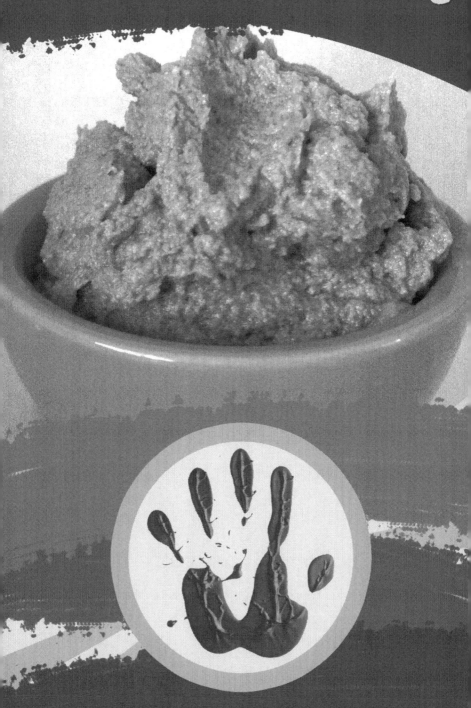

CHOCOLATE BUTTERCREAM FROSTING RECIPE

Frosting is a tricky item in the Paleo world. The point of frosting is to douse the pastry in super-sweet fluffy topping. But you can add flavor and texture to your cakes and cupcakes without adding refined sugars, and without smothering the delicious flavors of your pastry.

Ingredients:

- ½ cup coconut butter (coconut cream concentrate)
- ¼ cup coconut cream
- 1 tsp vanilla extract
- 2 tbsp raw honey, softened
- 1 tbsp cocoa powder (or more for dark chocolate)

Directions: Place all ingredients in the food processor and process until smooth. Store in an airtight container in the refrigerator up to one week.

Serving Size: 1/8 cup   Yields: 8 servings
Prep Time: 5 min   Total Time: 5 min

Coconut
Whipped Cream

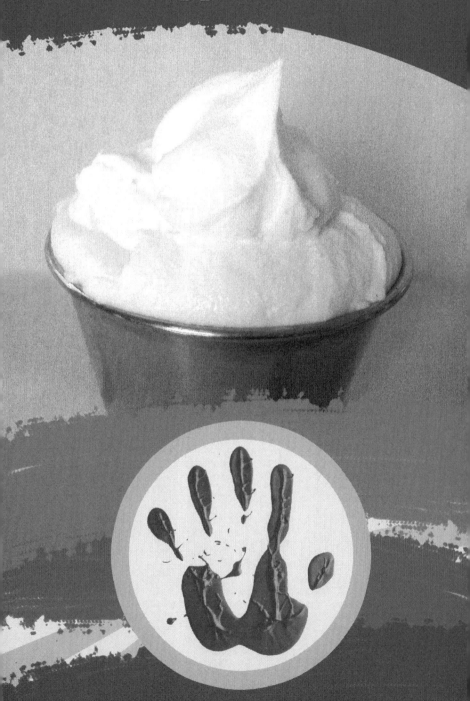

COCONUT WHIPPED CREAM RECIPE

Paleo coconut whipped cream is easier to make than the traditional dairy variety. Keep some in the fridge at all times. It's delicious on frozen mochas, cupcakes, ice cream, smoothies, pudding, and the list goes on. If you want to get crazy, spice it up with various extracts like peppermint, orange, or almond.

Ingredients:

- 1 14oz can full fat coconut milk
- 1 tbsp raw honey, melted but not hot
- ½ tsp vanilla extract

Directions: Place the can of coconut milk in the refrigerator upside down over night.

Flip the can right side up and poke a hole on either side of the lid with a can opener. Drain out the liquid. (You can save this! Coconut milk, yum!) Open the lid of the can and scoop the coconut cream into a mixing bowl. Whisk with a hand mixer or standing mixer until just fluffy. If you over mix it will "melt." Fold in the honey and vanilla extract.

Store in an airtight container in the refrigerator for up to one week. Allow to soften before serving. Keep in mind that the yield of this recipe will vary depending on the kind of coconut milk you use. Some have more fat, thus more cream, than other brands.

Serving Size: 2 tbsp   Yields: Varies
Prep Time: Overnight + 5 min   Total Time: Overnight + 5 min

NOTella

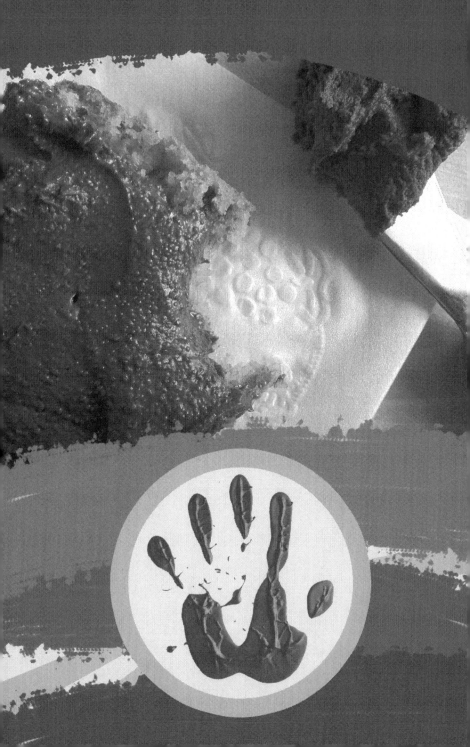

NOTELLA RECIPE

If you love the flavor of hazelnut with chocolate, your taste buds will jump for joy when you bite into a slice of banana bread (or toast, or apple slices, or anything) spread with this Paleo version of the popular Nutella.

Ingredients:

- 1 cup almond butter
- 1 cup hazelnut meal or shelled, roasted hazelnuts
- 4 tbsp raw honey
- 2 tbsp coconut oil
- 10 oz Paleo chocolate or extra dark chocolate, chunked

Directions: Place all ingredients in the food processor and process until smooth. Store in a jar in the refrigerator up to three weeks.

Serving Size: 2 tbsp   Yields: About 20 servings
Prep Time: 5 minutes   Total Time: 5 minutes

BEVERAGES

Frozen Mocha

~

Blender Hot Mocha Latte

Frozen Mocha

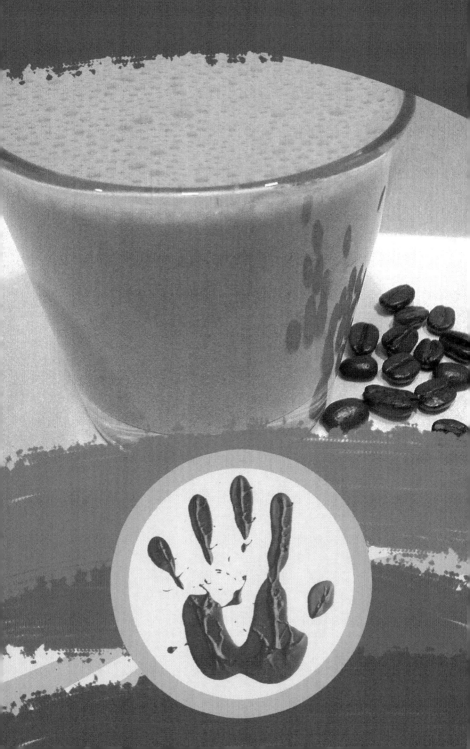

FROZEN MOCHA RECIPE

Better than a Frapped Coffee Drink and quicker than running to the local coffee shop, this frozen mocha will wake you and your taste buds up in the morning... or the afternoon. Feel free to adjust the coffee levels, add coconut whipped cream or a few sprigs of mint. Make it your way... this is just the beginning.

Ingredients:

- ½ cup cold coffee
- 1 cup coconut milk
- 1 frozen banana
- 5 ice cubes
- 3 tbsp cocoa powder
- 1 tsp vanilla extract
- Dash sea salt

Directions: Place all ingredients in your high-powered kitchen blender and process until smooth. Pour into a tall cup and enjoy. Try a dollop of coconut whipped cream on top!

Serving Size: 1 tall cup   Yields: 1 serving
Prep Time: 5 min   Total Time: 5 min

Blender Hot Mocha Latte

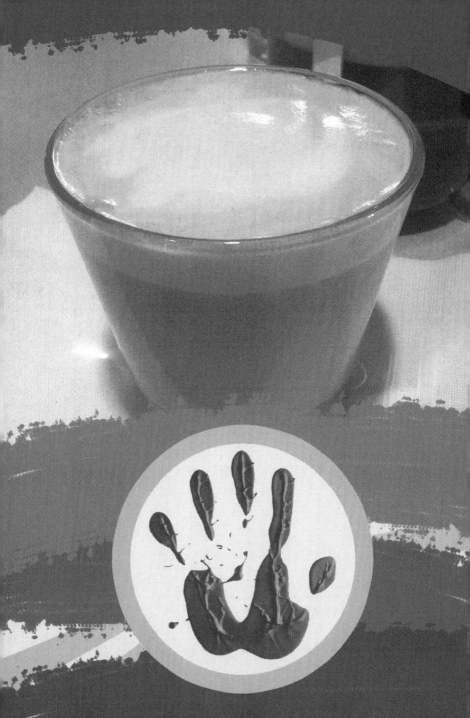

BLENDER HOT MOCHA LATTE RECIPE

Who needs a steaming wand when the blender works just fine? The key to making your morning mocha latte frothed on top is a high-powered kitchen blender, such as a Vitamix. It whirs so fast that it whips little air bubbles into the hot liquid, so when you pour, the froth rises... creamy and delicious.

Ingredients:

- 1 cup almond milk
- ½ cup hot strong coffee or espresso
- 3 tbsp cocoa powder (or to taste)
- 3 tbsp pure maple syrup (or birch xylitol)
- 1 tsp pure vanilla extract

Directions: Heat the almond milk in a small pot set over medium heat, about three minutes or until warm enough to suit your taste.

Place all ingredients in your high power kitchen blender set on high. Blend until frothy and smooth, about three minutes. Pour into a tall glass or mug and enjoy plain or with a dollop of coconut whipped cream.

Serving Size: 1 tall cup   Yields: 1 serving
Prep Time: 8 min   Total Time: 8 min

ABOUT THE AUTHOR

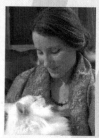

Kate Evans Scott is the author of the Amazon Bestselling cookbooks The Paleo Kid, Paleo Kid Snacks, The Paleo Kid Lunchbox, The Paleo Kid's Halloween, The Paleo Kid's Christmas and Infused: 26 Spa-Inspired Vitamin Waters.

After her son was diagnosed with several food intolerances and after having struggled with her own Autoimmune Disease, Kate made the commitment to remove all grains and processed foods from her family's diet. Her passion and love for good food blossomed after training with a retreat chef in Belgium in her early 20's. Since then, she has wanted to bring her love of food and health into the kitchens of other families struggling with health and dietary challenges.

Kate creates delicious dishes that are suitable for those suffering from digestive and autoimmune diseases - meals that nourish the body while healing the gut. Kate and her husband Mark live in Oregon with their two spirited children.

MORE BY KATE EVANS SCOTT

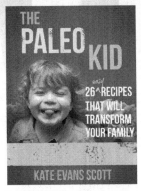

Available Now on Amazon

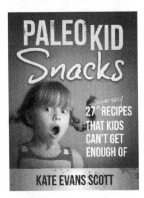

Available Now on Amazon

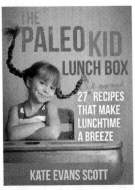

Available Now on Amazon

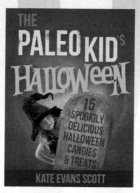

Available Now on Amazon

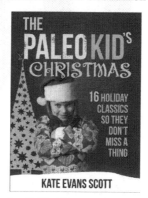

Available Now on Amazon

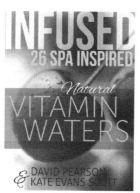

Available Now on Amazon

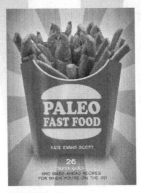
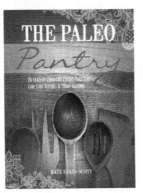

KATE EVANS SCOTT

RECIPE NOTES

RECIPE NOTES

Made in the USA
San Bernardino, CA
08 March 2017